HOW TO GET RID OF VAGINAL ODOR.

Exploring the best possible ways to sanitize the vaginal.

By

Dr DOUGLAS JASON

TABLE OF CONTENTS

TABLE OF CONTENTS

CHAPTER 7: WHEN IS IT TIME TO SEE A DOCTOR AND WHAT CAUSES VAGINAL DISCHARGE?

CONCLUSION

ABOUT THE AUTHOR

Dr DOUGLAS JASON is a certified dietician who has a strong passion for wellness and a big eagerness to help people all over the world. He uses healthy food, herbs, sauce and other useful tools to help mankind realized it's overall goal of optimum health.

INTRODUCTION

The vaginal area is usually somewhat scented. It is affected by diet and drink choices, cleanliness routines, and clothes. A stronger odor may also signal a medical concern that requires treatment.

Nutrition, health, and other variables may all have an impact on the natural scent of the vagina. Many products claim to "improve" vaginal odor, however, this is neither required nor safe.

Doing so may result in illnesses
that create or worsen an
unpleasant odor.

In this writing, we will look at ways
to reduce vaginal odor while also
treating any underlying medical
issues.

CHAPTER 1

VAGINAL ODOR.

Negative sentiments regarding vaginal odor might lead to self-esteem and body image issues.

It is common for the vagina to have a faint, musky odor.

This odor fluctuates as a result of hormonal changes throughout pregnancy, menopause, and the menstrual cycle. A faint odor is not the reason for the alarm.

Females who have different vaginal scents, on the other hand, should visit a doctor.

CHAPTER 2

TYPES OF VAGINAL ODOR.

<u>SMELL OF FISH</u>

When some events disrupt the intricate chemistry of the vagina, dangerous bacteria may proliferate uncontrollably, resulting in a fishy stench.

Bacterial vaginosis may induce this. This is the most prevalent vaginal infection in women aged 15 to 44.

Other symptoms of bacterial vaginosis in females include itching and burning. This may feel like a yeast infection. However, for many people, the fishy odor is the sole symptom.

Prescription medications may help cure an illness, and following certain healthy practices can limit the likelihood of recurrence. These are some examples:

Douches should be avoided since they might disrupt the delicate pH balance of the vagina.
Use of scented or flavored items in or around the vagina: Perfumes and other goods, such

as scented tampons, may affect vaginal chemistry and cause bacterial vaginosis.

Having fewer sexual partners and practicing safe sex: Although bacterial vaginosis is not a sexually transmitted illness (STI), having several sexual partners might disrupt the vaginal bacterial balance, possibly leading to bacterial vaginosis.

<u>ODOR OF SWEET OR BEER</u>

A yeast overgrowth in the vagina may give a pleasant odor akin to honey or cookies. Beer, flour, or bread may also be detected in the vagina. It might also have a sour odor at times.

Yeast infections are often accompanied by intense burning, itching, or symptoms of dryness. These symptoms usually worsen with time. Some ladies may also detect a cottage cheese-like discharge.

These illnesses can be managed with over-the-counter drugs. Females who have never had a yeast infection should contact a doctor to rule out other possibilities.

Many of the same precautions
that may be taken to prevent
bacterial vaginosis, such as
avoiding scented products and
never douching, can also be used
to prevent yeast overgrowth.

**Using antibiotics only when
necessary**: In certain females,
antibiotics might destroy healthy
vaginal bacteria, causing vaginal
yeast to proliferate.
**Not having oral intercourse with
someone who has thrush in
their mouth**: Thrush may be
spread by mouth-to-genital
contact.
**Maintaining a reasonably dry
vaginal area**: Because yeast

thrives in damp conditions, it is important to prevent leaving moisture on the vagina after washing. After a bath or shower, dry off with a towel and avoid sitting in damp swimwear or underwear.

Other smells

During menopause, hormonal changes may alter the fragrance of the vagina and leave it feeling dry.

Some STIs, most notably trichomoniasis, may also change the scent of the vagina.

Females should visit a doctor if they observe any changes in vaginal odor, especially if the odor is strong or unpleasant. They should not, however, apply perfume to cover the odor.

The parts that follow will provide some advice on how to avoid vaginal odor.

CHAPTER 3

TIPS TO REDUCE VAGINAL ODOR.

Embrace good hygiene methods. Vaginal odor may be reduced by using safe and gentle vaginal hygiene methods. Some pointers are as follows:

cleaning the vagina from front to back to prevent feces from entering the vagina

Urinating soon after sex, using a soft, fragrance-free soap on the vulva, merely changing underwear daily, or washing underwear in unscented products when sweaty or dirty

Taking a shower after sweating, since retained perspiration may exacerbate vaginal odor if there is an unpleasant odor, and gently wiping down the vulva with a washcloth between showers

Inserting soap into the vagina may change the pH of the vagina, thereby causing infections and an unpleasant odor.

Use menstruation products for internal use.

During menstruation, some women may detect a greater vaginal odor. Hormonal changes might produce an odor like iron or ammonia. Some menstruation products may trap odor, exacerbating the problem.

Use internal treatments to minimize vaginal odor caused by menstruation. The odor might be exacerbated by the wetness in maxi pads and reusable cotton pads. Sitting on a moist pad may potentially result in infection.

It is also essential to replace menstruation products regularly.

After sex, take care of your vagina.

Some individuals have a strong, fishy stench soon after sexual contact, which is an indication of bacterial vaginosis. Others may detect a less distinct odor.

Semen may mix with vaginal fluid and contribute to vaginal odor. Some lubricants may also change the pH of the vagina, affecting the fragrance.

CHAPTER 4:

A SIMPLE STEP TO REDUCE ODOR BEFORE AND AFTER VAGINAL INTERCOURSE.

To avoid contact between sperm and vaginal fluids, use a condom. Rinse the vulva under running water. Douching is not suggested by doctors.
Use scented or flavored lubricants sparingly.
Probiotics should be eaten up. Probiotics promote the growth of beneficial microorganisms throughout the human body,

including the vagina. They may also aid in the prevention of various vaginal infections, including yeast infections.

Probiotics may help restore the vagina's natural pH, lowering the likelihood of vaginal odor.

Evade unraveling apparel that is too tense.
Clothing may trap fluids and chemicals in and around the vagina, such as:

perspiration dead skin discharge previous intercourse sperm
Tight-fitting apparel, particularly certain shapewear, is often to

blame for trapping them. Fecal matter that enters the vagina may cause infections and smells, thus it is critical to avoid wearing clothes that promote its spread. Thong underwear is one example of this.

Breathable cotton is the ideal option for individuals concerned about vaginal odor since it is less prone to trap moisture around the vagina. This makes it more difficult for bacteria and other odor-causing agents to accumulate and generate a strong stink.

Lessen sugar and boost hydration

Consuming sugary meals may cause yeast overgrowth, which can exacerbate vaginal odor.

There is no study to support the usage of any particular diet to modify the scent of the vagina. Anecdotal data shows that eating sweet-smelling foods like watermelon, apple, and celery may assist.

Females should also make an effort to consume lots of water. Keeping hydrated helps to keep microorganisms at bay. It may help keep perspiration from smelling funny, resulting in a less noticeable vaginal odor.

CHAPTER 5

PRODUCTS THAT HELP REDUCE VAGINAL ODOR ARE DESCRIBED.

Probiotics

In certain circumstances, probiotics may help lessen vaginal odor. Probiotics, for example, have been shown in studies to lessen the symptoms of bacterial vaginosis. This is a disorder that causes a variety of vaginal symptoms, including odor.

Probiotics may be found in a variety of entire foods, including pickles, sauerkraut, kimchee, salsa, and several vegetables. Yogurts containing living cultures may also be a useful source of probiotics.

It is gluten-free and vegan-friendly.

It has three strands of 'good' bacteria, which include:

Lactobacillus acidophilus

L. rhamnosus B. lactis is less expensive per capsule than the next product, is appropriate for vegans, and does not contain gluten.

The FDA has no authority over the sale of probiotics or supplements.

Because the capsule includes gelatin, it is incompatible with vegans and vegetarians.

The Persona daily probiotic contains the following ingredients:

Acidophilus Blend (proprietary)

La-14 Lactobacillus acidophilus
SD-5857 Bifidobacterium bifidum
Ls-33 Lactobacillus salivarius
Lactobacillus bulgaricus Lb-87

Advantages

Persona's inexpensive pricing comprises five strains of "good" bacteria, and they produce their goods in the United States under stringent cGMP and FDA restrictions. They also provide worldwide delivery.

Cons: needs a Persona membership before purchasing; unclear if there is a minimum order quantity for this product. The FDA does not regulate the sale of probiotics or supplements that are more costly per capsule than the preceding product and are not suited for vegans or vegetarians.

According to the menstrual cup 2021 study, a menstrual cup may lessen odor when compared to other period items.

Size of Lena: little or huge
This item is available in two sizes: small and big. However, the firm advises that only experienced users buy the higher size.

Lena created this menstruation cup for teens as a beginner-friendly option. It is said to be soft silicone and may be worn for 12 hours straight.

According to the business, it is hypoallergenic, does not include latex, BPA, or dioxins, is biocompatible and safe throughout the production process, and is suited for beginners and teens.
three color options
Cons
Some reviews state that the product harmed them and caused them to suffer negative side effects.
Some reviewers also claim that the material is overly firm and that removing the cup was difficult.

It may take some time to become acclimated to menstruation cups.

It's constructed of super-soft silicone, which Saalt says is mild, flexible, and appropriate for individuals who have bladder sensitivity or who have pain with stiffer cups.

According to Saalt, it comprises 100% medical-grade silicone and colors that are non-irritating to the skin.

The cup may be worn for up to 12 hours.

Pros: Available in three vegan-friendly shades, Saalt provides 2% off every purchase to provide period care in underserved areas. includes a reinforced cuff to keep folds and leaks at bay incorporates grip rings to aid in the removal of the product

CHAPTER 6

PRODUCTS TO AVOID.

This section contains some examples of items that should be avoided while attempting to eliminate vaginal odor.

Douches

Using a douche in the vaginal region may help to erase odor temporarily. This, however, is not a long-term answer.

According to research, 29-92% of females globally douche in the vaginal region.

A modest 2019 research found that douching had no impact on vaginal odor for the majority of individuals.

Tampons and pads with fragrance

The ingredients in these scented sanitary products might aggravate an individual's vaginal odor.

According to research, scented vaginal deodorant products, such as scented tampons and pads, might cause discomfort and decrease vaginal health.

Soaps with scents

According to research, 29-92% of females globally douche in the vaginal region.

Using a douche in the vaginal region may help to erase odor temporarily. This, however, is not a long-term answer.

According to 2019 research, douching had no impact on vaginal odor for the majority of individuals.

According to research, scented vaginal deodorant items such as scented tampons and sanitary pads might cause discomfort and affect vaginal health.

Soaps with scents

According to the same study, using scented soaps might cause discomfort and infection in the vaginal region.

CHAPTER 7:

WHEN IS IT TIME TO SEE A DOCTOR AND WHAT CAUSES VAGINAL DISCHARGE?

If a person's vaginal odor does not improve after a few weeks, they should see a doctor.

Additionally, if a person has the following symptoms, in addition to vaginal odor, they should consult their doctor:

unexpected or increased vaginal discharge

vaginal discomfort, itching, or burning vaginal soreness urinating with a burning feeling. Vaginal odor is generally caused by a pH imbalance. This might occur as a result of an illness, age, sexual activity, or vaginal douching.

The usual vaginal pH ranges from 3.8 to 5.0, which is somewhat acidic. A higher pH may promote the growth of harmful bacteria, resulting in illness and potentially odor.

Clothing, hygiene practices, and specific meals and beverages might also contribute to vaginal odor.

It is natural for a woman to have a vaginal odor. However, if this stench becomes overpowering or smells strange, they may have an illness.

If the odor does not go away after a few weeks, it is recommended that a person contact a doctor. In addition, if they are experiencing additional symptoms in addition to vaginal odor, they should see a doctor.

CONCLUSION

Vaginal odor may be caused by a variety of causes, including food and drink, certain apparel, cleanliness, and diseases.

There are many strategies a person might take to counteract this vaginal odor. There are however certain things that should be avoided to lessen vaginal odor.

If a strange vaginal odor does not dissipate after a few weeks of attempting to erase it, the individual should see their doctor.